Copyri

Contents

What is Parkinson's disease?

Parkinson's disease is a nervous system disease that affects your ability to control movement. The disease usually starts out slowly and worsens over time. If you have Parkinson's disease, you may shake, have muscle stiffness, and have trouble walking and maintaining your balance and coordination. As the disease worsens, you may have trouble talking, sleeping, have mental and memory problems, experience behavioral changes and have other symptoms.

Who gets Parkinson's disease?

About 50% more men than women get Parkinson's disease. It is most commonly seen in persons 60 years of age and older. However, up to 10% of patients are diagnosed before age 50.

About 60,000 new cases of Parkinson's disease are diagnosed in the United States each year.

Is Parkinson's disease inherited?

Scientists have discovered gene mutations that are associated with Parkinson's disease.

There is some belief that some cases of early-onset Parkinson's disease – disease starting before age 50 – may be inherited. Scientists identified a gene mutation in people with Parkinson's disease whose brains contain Lewy bodies, which are clumps of the protein alpha-synuclein. Scientists are trying to understand the function of this protein and its relationship to genetic mutations that are sometimes seen in Parkinson's disease and in people with a type of dementia called Lewy body dementia.

Several other gene mutations have been found to play a role in Parkinson's disease. Mutations in these genes cause abnormal cell functioning, which affects the nerve cells' ability to release dopamine and causes nerve cell death. Researchers are still trying to discover what causes these genes to mutate in order to understand how gene mutations influence the development of Parkinson's disease.

Scientists think that about 10% to 15% of person's with Parkinson's disease may have a genetic mutation that predisposes them to development of the disease. There are also environmental factors involved that are not fully understood.

SYMPTOMS AND CAUSES

What causes Parkinson's disease?

Parkinson's disease occurs when nerve cells (neurons) in an area of the brain called the substantia nigra become impaired or die. These cells normally produce dopamine, a chemical (neurotransmitter) that helps the cells of the brain communicate (transmits signals, "messages," between areas in the brain). When these nerve cells become impaired or die, they produce less dopamine. Dopamine is especially important for the operation of another area of the brain called the basal ganglia. This area of the brain is responsible for organizing the brain's commands for body movement. The loss of dopamine causes the movement symptoms seen in people with Parkinson's disease.

People with Parkinson's disease also lose another neurotransmitter called norepinephrine. This chemical is needed for proper functioning of the sympathetic nervous system. This system controls some of the body's autonomic functions such as digestion, heart rate, blood pressure and breathing. Loss of norepinephrine causes some of the non-movement-related symptoms of Parkinson's disease.

Scientists aren't sure what causes the neurons that produce these neurotransmitter chemicals to die.

What are the symptoms of Parkinson's disease?

Symptoms of Parkinson's disease and the rate of decline vary widely from person to person. The most common symptoms include:

• Tremor: Shaking begins in your hands and arms. It can also occur in your jaw or foot. In the early stages of the disease, usually only one side of your body or one limb is affected. As the disease progresses, tremor may become more wide spread. It worsens with stress. Tremor often disappears during sleep and when your arm or leg is being moved.

• Slowness of movement (bradykinesia): This is the slowing down of movement and is caused by your brain's slowness in transmitting the necessary instructions to the appropriate parts of the body. This symptom is unpredictable and can be quickly disabling. One moment you may be moving easily, the next you may need help moving at all and finishing tasks such as getting dressed, bathing or getting out of a chair. You may even drag your feet as you walk.

• Rigid muscles/stiff limbs: Rigidity is the inability of your muscles to relax normally. This rigidity is caused by uncontrolled tensing of your muscles and results in you not being able to move about freely. You may experience aches or pains in the affected muscles and your range of motion may be limited.

• Unsteady walk and balance and coordination problems: You may develop a forward lean that makes you more likely to fall when bumped. You may take short shuffling steps, have difficulty starting to walk and difficulty stopping and not swing your arms naturally as you walk. You may feel like your feet are stuck to the floor when trying to take a step.

• Muscle twisting, spasms or cramps (dystonia). You may experience a painful cramp in your foot or curled and clenched toes. Dystonia can occur in other body parts.

• Stooped posture. You have a "hunched over" posture.

Other symptoms include:

• Decreased facial expressions: You may not smile or blink as often as the disease worsens; your face lacks expression.

• Speech/vocal changes: Speech may be quick, become slurred or be soft in tone. You may hesitate before speaking. The pitch of your voice may become unchanged (monotone).

• Handwriting changes: You handwriting may become smaller and more difficult to read.

• Depression and anxiety.

• Chewing and swallowing problems, drooling.

• Urinary problems.

• Mental "thinking" difficulties/memory problems.

• Hallucinations/delusions.

• Constipation.

• Skin problems, such as dandruff.

• Loss of smell.

- Sleeping disturbances including disrupted sleep, acting out your dreams, and restless leg syndrome.

- Pain, lack of interest (apathy), fatigue, change in weight, vision changes.

- Low blood pressure.

What are the different stages of Parkinson's disease?

Each person with Parkinson's disease experiences symptoms in in their own unique way. Not everyone experiences all symptoms of Parkinson's disease. You may not experience symptoms in the same order as others. Some people may have mild symptoms; others may have intense symptoms. How quickly symptoms worsen also varies from individual to individual and is difficult to impossible to predict at the outset.

In general, the disease progresses from early stage to mid-stage to mid-late-stage to advanced stage. This is what typically occurs during each of these stages:

Early stage

Early symptoms of Parkinson's disease are usually mild and typically occur slowly and do not interfere with daily activities. Sometimes early symptoms are not easy to detect or you may think early symptoms are simply normal signs of aging. You may have fatigue or a general sense of uneasiness. You may feel a slight tremor or have difficulty standing.

Often, a family member or friend notices some of the subtle signs before you do. They may notice things like body stiffness or lack of normal movement (no arm swing when walking) slow or small handwriting, lack of expression in your face, or difficulty getting out of a chair.

Mid stage

Symptoms start getting worse. Tremor, muscle stiffness and movement problems may now affect both sides of the body. Balance problems and falls are becoming more common. You may still be fully independent but daily tasks of everyday living, such as bathing and dressing, are becoming more difficult to do and take longer to complete.

Mid-late stage

Standing and walking are becoming more difficult and may require assistance with a walker. You may need full time help to continue to live at home.

Advanced stage

You now require a wheelchair to get around or are bedridden. You may experience hallucinations or delusions. You now require full-time nursing care.

DIAGNOSIS AND TESTS

How is Parkinson's disease diagnosed?

Diagnosing Parkinson's disease is sometimes difficult, since early symptoms can mimic other disorders and there are no specific blood or other laboratory tests to diagnose the disease.

Imaging tests, such as CT (computed tomography) or MRI (magnetic resonance imaging) scans, may be used to rule out other disorders that cause similar symptoms.

To diagnose Parkinson's disease, you will be asked about your medical history and family history of neurologic disorders as well as your current symptoms, medications and possible exposure to toxins. Your doctor will look for signs of tremor and muscle rigidity, watch you walk, check your posture and coordination and look for slowness of movement.

If you think you may have Parkinson's disease, you should probably see a neurologist, preferably a movement disorders-trained neurologist. The treatment decisions made early in the illness can affect the long-term success of the treatment.

MANAGEMENT AND TREATMENT

How is Parkinson's disease treated?

There is no cure for Parkinson's disease. However, medications and other treatments can help relieve some of your symptoms. Exercise can help your Parkinson's symptoms significantly. In addition, physical therapy, occupational therapy and speech-language therapy can help with walking and balance problems, eating and swallowing challenges and speech problems. Surgery is an option for some patients.

What medications are used to treat Parkinson's disease?

Medications are the main treatment method for patients with Parkinson's disease. Your doctor will work closely with you to develop a treatment plan best suited for you based on the severity of your disease at the time of diagnosis, side effects of the drug class and success or failure of symptom control of the medications you try.

Medications combat Parkinson's disease by:

• Helping nerve cells in the brain make dopamine.

• Mimicking the effects of dopamine in the brain.

• Blocking an enzyme that breaks down dopamine in the brain.

- Reducing some specific symptoms of Parkinson's disease.

Levodopa: Levodopa is a main treatment for the slowness of movement, tremor, and stiffness symptoms of Parkinson's disease. Nerve cells use levodopa to make dopamine, which replenishes the low amount found in the brain of persons with Parkinson's disease. Levodopa is usually taken with carbidopa (Sinemet®) to allow more levodopa to reach the brain and to prevent or reduce the nausea and vomiting, low blood pressure and other side effects of levodopa. Sinemet® is available in an immediate release formula and a long-acting, controlled release formula. Rytary® is a newer version of levodopa/carbidopa that is a longer-acting capsule. The newest addition is Inbrija®, which is inhaled levodopa. It is used by people already taking regular carbidopa/levodopa for when they have off episodes (discussed below).

As people have Parkinson's for a longer amount of time, the effects of their levodopa doses don't last as long as they did before, resulting in their symptoms (tremor, muscle rigidity, slowness) worsening before they are due to take their next dose. This is called 'wearing off.' They may also notice involuntary, fluid, dancing or fidgeting-like movements of their body called dyskinesias. These movements can indicate the levodopa dose is too high. These ups and downs of the effects of levodopa are called motor fluctuations and are often improve with adjustment of the medication by the neurologist.

Dopamine agonists: These drugs mimic the effects of dopamine in your brain. They are not as effective as levodopa in controlling slow muscle movement and muscle rigidity. Your doctor may try these medications first and add levodopa if your symptoms are not well controlled depending on severity of your symptoms and your age.

Newer dopamine medications include ropinirole (Requip®) and pramipexole (Mirapex®). Rotigotine (Neupro®) is given as a patch. Apomorphine (Apokyn®) is a short-acting injectable medication.

Side effects of dopamine agonists include nausea, vomiting, dizziness, lightheadedness, sleeping problems, leg swelling, confusion, hallucinations and compulsive behavior (such as excessive gambling, buying, eating, or sex). Some of these side effects are more likely to occur in people over 70 years old.

Catechol O-methyltransferase (COMT) inhibitors: These drugs block an enzyme that breaks down dopamine in your brain. These drugs are taken with levodopa and slow your body's ability to get rid of levodopa, so it lasts longer and is more reliable. Entacapone (Comtan®) and tolcapone (Tasmar®) are examples of COMT inhibitors. Opicapone (Ongentys®) is the newest medication in this class, receiving FDA approval in April 2020. Because these drugs increase the effectiveness of levodopa, they may also increase its side effects, including involuntary movements (dyskinesia). Tolcapone is rarely prescribed because it can damage the liver and requires close monitoring to prevent liver failure.

MAO B inhibitors. These drugs block a particular brain enzyme – monoamine oxidase B (MAO B) – that breaks down dopamine in your brain. This allows dopamine to have longer lasting effects on the brain. Examples of MAO B inhibitors include selegiline (Eldepryl®, Zelapar®), rasagiline (Azilect®) and safinamide (Xadago®). Side effects of these drugs include nausea and insomnia. Giving carbidopa-levodopa with an MAO B inhibitor increases the chance of hallucinations and dyskinesia. MAO B inhibitors are not prescribed if you are taking certain antidepressants or narcotic medications. Your doctor will review all your current medications and make the best treatment choice for you.

Anticholinergics. These drugs help reduce tremor and muscle stiffness. Examples include benztropine (Cogentin®) and trihexyphenidyl (Artane®). These are the oldest class of drugs to treat Parkinson's disease. Side effects include blurred vision, constipation, dry mouth and urine retention. Persons over age 70 who are prone to confusion and hallucinations or have memory impairment should not take anticholinergics. Because of the high rate of side effects these medications are less commonly used.

Amantadine. Amantadine (Symmetrel®), first developed as an antiviral agent, is useful in reducing the involuntary movements (dyskinesia) caused by levodopa medication. There are two extended-release forms of the drug, Gocovri®, and Osmolex ER®. Side effects include confusion and memory problems.

Istradefylline. Istradefylline (Nourianz®) is an adenosine A2A receptor antagonist. It is used for people taking carbidopa-levodopa but experiencing off symptoms. Like the other drugs that act to increase the effectiveness of levodopa, they may also increase its side effects, including involuntary movements (dyskinesia) and hallucinations.

What are the surgical treatments for Parkinson's disease?

Most patients with Parkinson's disease can maintain a good quality of life with medications. However, as the disease worsens, medications may no longer be effective in some patients. In these patients, the effectiveness of medications becomes unpredictable – reducing symptoms during "on" periods and no longer controlling symptoms during "off" periods, which usually occur when the medication is wearing off and just before the next dose is to be taken. Sometimes these variations can be managed with changes in medications. However, sometimes they can't. Based on the type and severity of your symptoms, the failure of adjustments in your medications, the decline in your quality of life and your overall health, your doctor may discuss some of the available surgical options.

• Deep brain stimulation (DBS) involves implanting electrodes in the brain, which deliver electrical impulses that block or change the abnormal activity that cause symptoms. DBS can treat most of the major movement symptoms of Parkinson's disease such as tremor, slowness of movement (bradykinesia) and stiffness (rigidity). It does not improve memory, hallucinations, depression, and the other non-movement symptoms of Parkinson's disease. Only patients whose symptoms are not controlled despite medication trials and who meet other strict criteria may be candidates for DBS. Your doctor will discuss if this is the right treatment for you.

- Carbidopa-levodopa infusion involves the surgical placement of a feeding tube into the small intestine. A gel form of the medication carbidopa-levodopa (Duopa®) is delivered through this tube. This method of continuous infusion of the drug keeps a stable dosage in the body. This helps patients who have had variation in their response to the oral form of carbidopa-levodopa but are still benefitting from the combination drug.

• Pallidotomy involves destroying a small portion of a part of the brain that controls movement (the globus pallidus). Pallidotomy help reduce involuntary movements (dyskinesias), muscle stiffness and tremor.

• Thalamotomy involves destroying a small part of the thalamus. This may help a small number of patients who have severe tremors of their arm or hand.

PREVENTION

Can Parkinson's disease be prevented?

Unfortunately, no. Parkinson's disease is long-term disease that worsens over time. Although there is no way to prevent or cure the disease (at this current moment in time), medications may significantly relieve your symptoms. In some patients – especially those with later-stage disease, surgery to improve symptoms may be an option.

OUTLOOK / PROGNOSIS

What is the outlook for persons with Parkinson's disease?

Although there is no cure or absolute evidence of ways to prevent Parkinson's disease, scientists are working hard to learn more about the disease and find innovative ways to better manage it, prevent it from progressing and ultimately curing it.

Currently, you and your healthcare team's efforts are focused on medical management of your symptoms along with general health and lifestyle improvement recommendations (exercise, healthy eating, improved sleep). By identifying individual symptoms and adjusting the course of action based on changes in symptoms, most people with Parkinson's disease can live fulfilling lives.

The future is hopeful. Some of the research underway includes:

• Using stem cells (from either bone marrow or embryos) to produce new neurons, which would produce dopamine.

• Producing a dopamine-producing enzyme that is delivered to a gene in the brain that controls movement.

• Using a naturally occurring human protein – glial cell-line derived neurotrophic factor, GDNF – to protect dopamine-releasing nerve cells.

Many other investigations are underway too. Much has been learned, much progress has been made and additional discoveries are likely to come.

LIVING WITH

What lifestyle changes can I make to ease Parkinson's symptoms?

Exercise: Exercise helps improve muscle strength, balance, coordination, flexibility, and tremor. It is also strongly believed to improve memory, thinking and reduce the risk of falls and decrease anxiety and depression. One study in persons with Parkinson's disease showed that 2.5 hours of exercise per week resulted in improved ability to move and a slower decline in quality of life compared to those who didn't exercise or didn't start until later in the course of their disease. Some exercises to consider include strengthening or resistance training, stretching exercises or aerobics (running, walking, dancing). All types of exercise are helpful.

Eat a healthy, balanced diet: This is not only good for your general health but can ease some of the non-movement related symptoms of Parkinson's, such as constipation. Eating foods high in fiber in particular can relieve constipation. The Mediterranean diet is one example of a healthy diet.

Preventing falls and maintaining balance: Falls are a frequent complication of Parkinson's. While you can do many things to reduce your risk of falling, the two most important are: 1) to work with your doctor to ensure that your treatments — whether medicines or deep brain stimulation — are optimal; and 2) to consult with a physical therapist who can assess your walking and balance. The physical therapist is the expert when it comes to recommending assistive devices or exercise to improve safety and preventing falls.

Improve the quality of your sleep.

How do I prevent falls from common hazards?

- Floors: Remove all loose wires, cords, and throw rugs. Minimize clutter. Make sure rugs are anchored and smooth. Keep furniture in its usual place.

- Bathroom: Install grab bars and non-skid tape in the tub or shower. Use non-skid bath mats on the floor or install wall-to-wall carpeting.

- Lighting: Make sure halls, stairways, and entrances are well-lit. Install a night light in your bathroom or hallway and staircase. Turn lights on if you get up in the middle of the night. Make sure lamps or light switches are within reach of the bed if you have to get up during the night.

• Kitchen: Install non-skid rubber mats near the sink and stove. Clean spills immediately.

• Stairs: Make sure treads, rails, and rugs are secure. Install a rail on both sides of the stairs. If stairs are a threat, it might be helpful to arrange most of your activities on the lower level to reduce the number of times you must climb the stairs.

• Entrances and doorways: Install metal handles on the walls adjacent to the doorknobs of all doors to make it more secure as you travel through the doorway.

What are some tips to help me maintain balance?

• Keep at least one hand free at all times. Try using a backpack or fanny pack to hold things rather than carrying them in your hands. Never carry objects in both hands when walking as this interferes with keeping your balance.

• Attempt to swing both arms from front to back while walking. This might require a conscious effort if Parkinson's disease has diminished your movement. It will, however, help you to maintain balance and posture, and reduce falls.

• Consciously lift your feet off of the ground when walking. Shuffling and dragging of the feet is a common culprit in losing your balance.

• When trying to navigate turns, use a "U" technique of facing forward and making a wide turn, rather than pivoting sharply.

• Try to stand with your feet shoulder-length apart. When your feet are close together for any length of time, you increase your risk of losing your balance and falling.

• Do one thing at a time. Don't try to walk and accomplish another task, such as reading or looking around. The decrease in your automatic reflexes complicates motor function, so the less distraction, the better.

• Do not wear rubber or gripping soled shoes-- they might "catch" on the floor and cause tripping.

• Move slowly when changing positions. Use deliberate, concentrated movements and, if needed, use a grab bar or walking aid. Count 15 seconds between each movement. For example, when rising from a seated position, wait 15 seconds after standing to begin walking.

• If you become "frozen," visualize stepping over an imaginary object, or have someone place his or her foot in front of yours to step over. Try not to have a caregiver or family member "pull" you--this might throw you off balance and even prolong the episode.

• If balance is a continuous problem, you might want to consider a walking aid such as a cane, walking stick, or walker. Once you've mastered walking with help, you might be ready to try it on your own again.

How Does Parkinson's Disease Change the Way You Eat?

If you've been diagnosed with Parkinson's disease, you may have noticed some changes in your appetite and eating habits, says Dr. Subramanian.

For example, some of your prescription medications may work best on an empty stomach, but they may also cause nausea in some people when taken without food.

"We advise people to take their medication about an hour before meals, if possible, to avoid any protein interaction," Subramanian says. Eating protein-rich foods like meat, fish, eggs, dairy products, nuts, and beans too close to the time you take medications can interfere with how the body processes some medications prescribed to treat Parkinson's disease, which may cause them to work less quickly or less effectively.

If you experience nausea after taking your medication on an empty stomach, your doctor may recommend eating a small, light snack like crackers or applesauce before taking your pills.

Subramanian also notes that loss of appetite and subsequent weight loss are a major concern for people with Parkinson's disease. This may be caused by symptoms such as difficulty swallowing, decreased ability to taste or smell, nausea side effects from medications, or movement problems (with your hands and wrists) that make it difficult to eat.

To address these issues, the Parkinson's Foundation recommends:

• Placing dishes on rubber mats to prevent them from slipping while eating

• Using weighted utensils — for example, the "Parkinson's spoon" — and cups

• Using cups with lids or straws to reduce spilling

• Cutting foods into smaller pieces and chewing extensively to ease swallowing

• Eating foods that are easier to swallow, such as soups and pureed dishes

• Eating bitter green vegetables like kale or spinach or spicy foods to stimulate your appetite and add taste to food

• Exercising before meals to increase hunger

How a "Parkinson's Spoon" Can Make Eating and Drinking Easier

Parkinson's disease symptoms like tremor, joint stiffness, or difficulty swallowing may make eating certain foods challenging. Try consulting an occupational therapist, who can recommend assistive devices that will make eating and drinking easier, says Subramanian.

One option: Use a "Parkinson's spoon." This popular device is designed to make mealtime easier for people with Parkinson's disease. There are different products available, but all of them are eating utensils that have been equipped with a special design or technology that helps stabilize them as you eat.

Dietitians, Speech Pathologists, and Mental Health Experts Can Help, Too

Talking to a registered dietitian can help you make changes to your diet — for example, by learning how to use thickening liquids or soften solid foods.

If swallowing continues to be a problem, a speech-language pathologist may be able to help you find ways to make swallowing easier.

"A speech pathologist who is also a swallow therapist can do a swallow study, a test during which you try different foods and they monitor how you swallow using an X-ray machine," Subramanian explains. "Food aspiration, or when food gets into your lungs, can be a problem with Parkinson's disease, so the swallow study can identify problem foods and your doctors can recommend changes and diet modifications to make eating safer."

Finally, as anxiety or depression are common in people with Parkinson's and can suppress appetite, it's important to recognize symptoms associated with these behavioral health conditions and seek out treatment if needed.

Parkinson's disease," Subramanian adds. "So in some cases, we recommend a little extra salt in the diet, or even energy drinks, to boost blood pressure."

Either way, you should check with your doctor about taking appropriate dietary steps to manage blood pressure along with Parkinson's disease.

Also limit foods high in calories and fat, particularly saturated and trans fat, which can increase your risk of heart problems as well as certain types of cancer and make it more difficult for you maintain a healthy weight.

It's important to balance what you eat with your level of physical activity — meaning: if you don't exercise much because of your Parkinson's disease symptoms, you need to watch how many calories you're consuming.

Speaking of calories, alcoholic beverages add a lot, while providing your body with few (if any) nutrients. Plus, drinking alcohol can increase your risk of accidents and falls. Best to avoid alcohol altogether, but if you do choose to imbibe, first check with your doctor about possible interactions between liquor and your medications.

Eating Right With Parkinson's Disease

You don't need to follow a special diet if you have Parkinson's disease. But the condition, which makes your body movements stiff or tough to control, can make it harder for you to eat well. But you need nutritious foods to keep up your strength and to make sure your Parkinson's meds work as they're supposed to.

It's common for people with Parkinson's to lose weight, have trouble swallowing and pooping, and feel nauseated from medications. Your doctor or a registered dietitian may be able to offer advice on the best ways to handle those issues.

How to Eat Well

Eat a variety of foods from each food category, like fruits, vegetables, and lean meats. If you think you need vitamin supplements, check with your doctor first.

Keep your weight in the healthy range for your age and height with exercise and a good diet.

Load up on fiber with foods like broccoli, peas, apples, cooked split peas and beans, whole-grain breads, cereals, and pasta.

Cut down on sugar, salt, and saturated fats from meat and dairy, and cholesterol.

Drink 8 cups of water every day.

Ask your doctor you can drink alcohol. It may keep your medications from working right.

Taking Your Drugs and Food Together

Levodopa is the best medication for Parkinson's. Ideally, you should take it on an empty stomach, about 30 minutes before eating or at least one hour after a meal. But that can cause nausea in some people. Your doctor may prescribe something else or a different mix of drugs, which may not always make the nausea go away. In that case, your doctor may recommend you take medication for your side effects.

Also, ask your doctor if you should cut down on protein. In rare cases, a high-protein diet can make levodopa work less well.

Control Nausea

To prevent or relieve nausea, try these tips:

- Stick to clear or ice-cold drinks. Sugary drinks may calm your stomach better than other liquids.
- Avoid orange and grapefruit juices and other acidic beverages.
- Sip slowly.
- Drink liquids between meals instead of during them.
- Eat bland foods like saltine crackers or plain bread.
- Avoid fried, greasy, or sweet foods.
- Eat slowly, and eat smaller, more frequent meals.
- Don't mix hot and cold foods.

- Eat cold or room-temperature foods to avoid getting nauseated from the smell of hot or warm foods.

- Rest after eating, but keep your head upright. Activity may worsen nausea and may make you vomit.

- Don't brush your teeth after eating.

- If you wake up feeling nauseated, eat some crackers before you hop out of bed. Before bedtime, try a high-protein snack like lean meats or cheese.

- Try to eat when you're less nauseated.

Thirst or Dry Mouth

Some Parkinson's medications may make you feel parched. You might try these tips for relief:

Drink at least 8 cups of liquid each day. Some people with Parkinson's also have heart problems and may need to watch their fluid levels. Check with your doctor about how much you need to drink.

Limit caffeine from coffee, tea, cola, and chocolate as it can interfere with some of your meds and make you thirstier.

Soften breads, toast, cookies, or crackers. You can dunk them in milk or decaffeinated tea or coffee.

Sip a drink after each bite of food to moisten your mouth and help you swallow.

Add sauces to foods to make them soft and moist. Try gravy, broth, sauce, or melted butter.

Eat sour candy or fruit ice to help make more saliva and moisten your mouth.

Stay away from most mouthwashes, which often contain alcohol that can dry your mouth. Ask your doctor or dentist if there's anything else you should do.

Ask your doctor about prescription artificial saliva.

Eating When You're Tired

If you don't have energy for meals later in the day, you can:

Pick foods that are easy to fix, and save your energy for eating. If you live with your family, let them help you make your meal.

Look into a delivery service. Some grocery stores have them. Or you can check if you might be able to get food delivered from your local Meals on Wheels program for free or for a small fee.

Keep healthy snack foods on hand, like fresh fruit and vegetables or high-fiber cold cereals.

Freeze extra portions of what you cook so you have a quick meal when you feel worn out.

Rest before you eat so you can enjoy your meal. And eat your biggest meal early in the day to fuel yourself for later.

When You Have No Appetite

Some days, you just may not feel like eating at all.

Talk to your doctor. Sometimes, depression can cause poor appetite. Your hunger likely will return when you get treatment.

Walk or do another light activity to rev up your appetite.

Drink beverages after you've finished eating so you don't feel full before the meal.

Include your favorite foods in your menu. Eat the high-calorie foods on your plate first. But avoid empty calories from sugary sodas, candies, and chips.

Perk up your meals by trying different dishes and ingredients.

Choose high-protein and high-calorie snacks, including:

- Ice cream

- Cheese

- Granola bars

- Custard

- Sandwiches

- Nachos with cheese

- Eggs

- Crackers with peanut butter

- Cereal with half and half

- Greek yogurt

Stay at a Healthy Weight

Malnutrition and weight loss are often problems for people with Parkinson's. So it's good to keep track of your weight.

Weigh yourself once or twice a week, unless your doctor says to do it more often. If you are taking diuretics or steroids, such as prednisone, you should step on the scale daily.

If you gain or lose weight noticeably (2 pounds in a day or 5 pounds in a week), talk to your doctor. They may want change your food and drinks to manage your condition.

If you need to gain weight:

Ask your doctor if nutritional supplements are right for you. Some can be harmful or interfere with your medication.

Avoid low-fat or low-calorie foods unless you've been told otherwise. Instead, use whole milk, whole milk cheese, and yogurt.

Foods to eat

The following foods may be beneficial for slowing disease progression or for lowering the risk of Parkinson's disease.

Foods containing nutrients that people may be deficient in

Some researchTrusted Source suggests that people with Parkinson's often have certain nutrient deficiencies, including deficiencies in iron, vitamin B1, vitamin C, zinc, and vitamin D.

The above study points out that some of these deficiencies may be associated with neuroinflammation and neurodegeneration, which are key factors in Parkinson's.

Therefore, people with Parkinson's may wish to consume more of the following foods.

Foods containing iron

The following foods are good sources of iron:

- liver

- red meat

- beans

- nuts

Foods containing vitamin B1

The following foods are good sources of vitamin B1:

- peas

- bananas

- oranges

- nuts

- wholegrain bread

Foods containing vitamin C

The following foods are good sources of vitamin C:

- citrus fruits

- peppers

- strawberries

- broccoli

- potatoes

Foods containing zinc

The following foods are good sources of zinc:

- meat

- shellfish

- bread

- cereal products, such as wheat germ

Foods containing vitamin D

The following foods are good sources of vitamin D:

- oily fish

- red meat

- egg yolks

- certain fortified foods

Antioxidants

Current research focuses on proteinsTrusted Source, flavonoids, and gut bacteriaTrusted

Source for improving Parkinson's symptoms. In the meantime, eating a diet high in antioxidants reduces "oxidative stress" that aggravates Parkinson's and similar conditions, according to the Michael J. Fox Foundation for Parkinson's research.

You can get lots of antioxidants by eating:

• tree nuts, like walnuts, Brazil nuts, pecans, and pistachios

• blueberries, blackberries, goji berries, cranberries, and elderberries

• tomatoes, peppers, eggplant, and other nightshade vegetables

• spinach and kale

Eating a plant-based diet high in these types of foods may provide the highest antioxidant intake.

Clinical trials over the last decade explored the idea of antioxidant treatment for Parkinson's, but these trials didn't find concrete evidence to link antioxidants to Parkinson's treatment. But decreasing oxidative stress is still a simple way to improve your lifestyle and get healthier. In other words, it can't hurt.

Fava beans

Some people eat fava beans for Parkinson's because they contain levodopa — the same ingredient in some drugs used to treat Parkinson's. There's no definitive evidence supporting fava beans as a treatment at this time. Since you don't know how much levodopa you're getting when you eat fava beans, they can't substitute for prescription treatments.

Omega-3s

If you're concerned about secondary symptoms of Parkinson's, like dementia and confusion, get serious about consuming more salmon, halibut, oysters, soybeans, flax seed, and kidney beans. SoyTrusted Source in particular is being studied for its ability to protect against Parkinson's. These foods contain omega-3 fatty acids, which might improveTrusted Source cognitive function.

A healthy diet in general

While the above foods may be beneficial for people with Parkinson's, it is most important for people with Parkinson's to focus on their diet as a whole.

The Parkinson's Foundation suggest that people with Parkinson's follow these dietary tips:

• Avoid fad diets and try to consume foods from all food groups.

• Consume plenty of grains, vegetables, and fruits.

• Limit sugar intake.

• Reduce salt and sodium intake.

• Consume foods that contain antioxidants, such as brightly colored and dark fruits and vegetables.

• Follow a diet that is low in fat, saturated fat, and cholesterol.

• Drink alcohol only in moderation.

Foods to avoid

Foods that are hard to chew

Many people with Parkinson's have difficulty with chewing and swallowing foods. A person needs medical help if this is the case. A speech and language therapist may be able to help a person overcome this issue.

However, if a person is finding certain foods hard to chew and swallow, they may wish to avoid these foods.

Such foods include:

• hard foods

- dry, crumbly foods

- tough or chewy meats

If a person does wish to eat chewy meats, they could try using gravy or sauce to soften them and make eating easier.

They could also try chopping meat into smaller pieces or incorporating meat into casseroles, which can make it more tender.

Having a drink with a meal can also make chewing and swallowing easier.

Dairy products

Dairy products have been linkedTrusted Source to a risk of developing Parkinson's. Something in dairy products might negatively impact the oxidation levels in your brain, making symptoms more persistent. This effect was shown to be stronger in men than in women and not seen in those supplementing with calcium.

If you're going to stop consuming dairy products like milk, cheese, and yogurt, you might want to consider a calcium supplement to make up for the loss of calcium in your diet. However, low calcium intake doesn't necessarily equal poor bone health, as seen in countries with low dairy and calcium consumption.

Recent research suggests that a defect in how the body manages calcium ions (Ca^{2+}), the form of calcium residing in bone, and also present in dairy, might be to blame for the progression of Parkinson's disease.

Foods high in saturated fat

The role that foods high in saturated fats play in Parkinson's progression is still under investigationTrusted Source and is often conflicting. We might eventually discover that there are certain types of saturated fats that actually help people with Parkinson's.

Some limited research does show that ketogenic, low-protein diets were beneficial for some with Parkinson's. Other research finds high saturated fat intake worsened risk.

But in general, foods that have been fried or heavily processed alter your metabolism, increase blood pressure, and impact your cholesterol. None of those things are good for your body, especially if you're trying to treat Parkinson's.

Processed foods

Some studies suggest that eating a "Western-style" diet may be linked with symptom severity in Parkinson's.

This type of diet is high in processed foods. Some examples of processed foods include:

• canned foods

• sodas

• breakfast cereals

• chips

• bacon

• ready meals

- candy

- cakes

One study suggests that several of these items, including canned foods and sodas, may be associated with "more rapid [Parkinson's] progression."

Also, the researcher behind another study points out that eating a lot of processed foods "contributes to increased intestinal permeability and dysbiosis due to an overgrowth of gram-negative bacteria."

Lifestyle tips

Staying hydrated is important for everyone, especially people with Parkinson's. Aim to drink six to eight glasses of water each day to feel your best.

Vitamin D has been demonstrated to protect against Parkinson's, so getting fresh air and sunshine might help your symptoms, too. Different kinds of exercise and physical therapy can improve your abilities and slow the progression of Parkinson's.

Talk to you doctor about supplements you might take and exercises that would be safe for you to try.

Combine exercise with diet

If you want to feel your best, combine a healthy diet with exercise. Research has shown that regular exercise can improve PD symptoms.

"Do exercise that raises your heart rate," Dr. Gostkowski says. "Aim for about 30 minutes a day, five days a week." Don't worry about specific exercises. Do an activity you enjoy, as long as it gets your heart rate up. Try brisk walking or biking or more advanced exercise for veteran athletes. "I recommend seeing an occupational therapist. They can tailor an exercise program to your needs."

What types of exercise can help manage Parkinson's disease?

There are several types of exercises you can do to manage Parkinson's disease. You can create a varied routine based on your specific concerns, fitness level, and overall health.

Aim to do at least a few minutes of movement each day. Include exercises that improve cardiovascular health, flexibility, and strength. If you change up your exercises every week. your body can learn new ways to move.

There are a few different types of exercise that may be especially helpful to those with Parkinson's, including:

• physical and occupational therapy

• yoga

• aerobics

Best physical and occupational therapy exercises

Physical therapy exercises target your areas of concern. They can help develop your strength, balance, and coordination. You'll also enhance your functional mobility by improving concentration, flexibility, and range of motion.

Occupational therapy exercises are intended to help you perform daily activities related to work, school, or home with greater ease.

Single leg stand

This exercise helps to improve standing balance and ability to walk. It also develops steadiness, strength, and confidence.

For support, rest your hands on a wall or the back of a chair.

1. Place your weight on your less dominant leg.

2. Slowly lift your opposite foot from the floor.

3. Hold for 20 seconds. Try to use your arms as little as possible for balance.

4. Lower your foot to the floor.

5. Repeat on the other side.

Wrist curls

Hand exercises help to increase steadiness, reduce tremors, and improve finger and hand dexterity.

For this exercise, use a dumbbell that's 1 to 5 pounds.

1. Place your left hand and wrist over the edge of a table with your palm facing up.

2. Hold the weight in your hand.

3. Slowly move your wrist up as far as you can.

4. Hold this position for a few seconds.

5. Do 1 to 2 sets of 12 repetitions.

6. Repeat on the opposite side.

Best yoga poses

Yoga exercises develop balance, improve flexibility, and enhance concentration. They also help with body awareness mindfulness. Yoga has a positive effect on breathing, and it helps to promote relaxation.

A small 2018 study found that people with Parkinson's disease who did yoga twice weekly for 8 weeks significantly reduced their fall risk compared to the control group. The yoga group also showed improvements in posture stability, as well as functional and freezing gait.

Child's pose (Balasana)

This gentle forward bend relieves mental and physical tiredness and promotes a sense of inner calm. It also loosens up your hips, thighs, and ankles. Plus, it relieves back tightness and discomfort.

For extra support, place a cushion under your forehead, torso, or bottom.

1. Sit back on your heels with your knees together or slightly apart.

2. Hinge at your hips to fold forward.

3. Extend your arms in front of you or rest your arms alongside your body.

4. Place your forehead on the floor or a cushion.

5. Relax deeply, letting go of any tension in your body.

6. Hold this pose for up to 5 minutes.

Warrior II (Virabhadrasana II)

This stamina-building pose improves balance while stretching and strengthening your body.

1. From standing, step your left foot back and turn your toes to the left at a slight angle.

2. Keep your right toes facing forward and open your hips to the side.

3. Raise your arms so they're parallel to the floor, turning your palms down.

4. Bend your right knee until it's behind or above your ankle.

5. Press into both feet, elongate your spine, and feel a line of energy moving from your front to back fingertips.

6. Gaze ahead toward the tip of your middle finger.

7. Hold this position for up to 1 minute.

8. Repeat on the opposite side.

Modifications:

• Place a chair under your front thigh.

• Position yourself alongside a wall, leaning into it as needed.

• Lower your back knee to the floor.

• Position your feet closer together.

Best aerobic exercises

Aerobic exercises improve flexibility, enhance mobility, and build strength. They boost your cardiovascular health and lung function while burning calories.

Research from 2020 points to the effectiveness of aerobic exercise in improving physical fitness and motor symptoms in people with Parkinson's disease. Larger, more in-depth studies examining the long-term benefits of aerobic exercise are needed.

No-contact boxing

This activity improves strength, speed, and agility. It also increases endurance, balance, and hand-eye coordination.

To learn no-contact boxing, join a class at your local fitness center, hire a private teacher, or try the moves described below.

Jab punches

1. Stand with your feet under your hips, or slightly wider for better balance.

2. Make fists and place them in front of your shoulders with your palms facing forward.

3. Punch your left fist forward, extending your arm fully.

4. Return to the starting position.

5. Repeat on the opposite side.

6. This is one repetition.

7. Do 1 to 2 sets of 20 repetitions.

Add medication for a winning combo

Diet and exercise are important for managing PD, but don't forget about medications. Take them regularly and exactly as your doctor prescribes.

If you tend to forget your medication, set an alarm to remind you. You can also use a pillbox that's labeled with days and times of day. "Take your meds on a set schedule, don't skip doses and don't double dose," says Dr. Gostkowski. "When you're diligent about taking your medications and following a healthy lifestyle, you'll feel your best."

Sample Meal Plan

Day 1:

For people using levodopa

*NOTE: Take levodopa 30–60 minutes before eating.

Breakfast

– Whole-grain hot cereal such as oatmeal, cooked barley flakes, or Seven-Grain Cereal

– Milk (if sensitive to milk protein, choose a milk alternative such as almond, soy, or rice milk)

– Fruit juice (unsweetened)

– Coffee or tea

Protein-free snack

– Water kefir

– Two portions of fresh fruit (banana, grapes, chopped pineapple, sliced oranges, kiwifruit or other fruit of choice)

Lunch

- Sandwich on whole-grain bread, sliced turkey, cheese, lettuce, mayonnaise

- Devilled egg

- Deli-style fermented pickle

- Milk, milk alternative or fruit juice

- Coffee or tea

Low-protein snack

- A handful of peanuts or roasted cashew nuts

Evening meal

- Miso soup

-Stir-fry of shrimp, snow peas, carrot, mushroom and onion

- Kimchi

– Brown rice

– Soy sauce

– Dates or figs

Day 2:

Breakfast

– Fried or poached egg

– Sausage patty

– Whole-wheat toast with butter

– Yoghurt with sliced banana

– Fruit juice

– Coffee or tea

Low-protein or protein-free snack

– Smoothie made with fruit and a milk alternative (almond milk, etc.)

– Rye or whole-grain cracker with peanut butter

Lunch

– Lentil or split pea soup

– Whole-grain crackers

– Cheese

– Mediterranean olives

– Vegetable juice

– Coffee or tea

Protein-free snack

– Popcorn

Evening meal

– Grilled salmon

– Cooked quinoa or baked potato with butter

– Asparagus

– Sliced tomato

– Sauerkraut

– Whole-grain dinner roll

– Cantaloupe half

Day 3:

For people using rasagiline

*Note: All vegetables and fruits should be fresh, not overripe; meat, poultry and fish should be fresh, not aged or smoked, or else canned or frozen and eaten immediately after opening or thawing. Eggs, cooked dried beans, peas, and small quantities of nuts and peanut butter are safe. Avoid aged cheeses and meats and foods containing meat extracts such as bouillon or beef broth, fermented soy products such as tofu, soy sauce and miso, other fermented foods except for yoghurt, which is safe. Since fermented foods are limited, you may wish to consider a probiotic supplement, such as gelcaps. See also my tyramine booklet for more information.

Breakfast

– Oatmeal with milk

– Orange juice (fresh, or frozen and reconstituted)

– Coffee or tea

Snack

– Whole-wheat blueberry muffin with butter

Lunch

– Tuna salad sandwich on whole-wheat bread

– Raw carrot, celery, radishes

– Fresh milk, vegetable juice, coffee or tea

Snack

– Plain yoghurt, with sliced banana and honey

Evening meal

– Beef steak (fresh, not aged)

– Brussels sprouts, lightly steamed with fresh lemon juice

– Baked sweet potato with butter and honey

– Whole-grain dinner roll with butter

– Baked apple with maple syrup

Day 4:

Breakfast

– Eggs (cooked as you like)

– Fresh sausage

– Whole-wheat toast with butter

– Mixed berry compote (fresh, or thawed from frozen)

– Coffee or tea

Snack

– Cottage cheese, cantaloupe

Lunch

Vegetable soup (made with fresh ingredients including legumes, but no aged meats or meat extracts)

– Whole-grain crackers

– Fresh milk, vegetable juice, coffee or tea

Snack

– Yoghurt smoothie with banana and honey

Evening meal

– Grilled shrimp with whole-grain linguine, extra-virgin olive oil, garlic

– Fresh spinach salad

¬– Roasted carrots

– Whole-grain garlic bread

– A few pieces of dark chocolate

PARKINSON'S DIET RECIPES

Trying parkinson-friendly recipes is a great way to explore new flavors and find new favorite dishes while looking after your health. In this part are nourishing parkinson's diet recipes for you to enjoy and manage your symptoms.

Blue Majik Pancakes

Preparation time

12 minutes

Ingredients

- 1 cup of almond flour

- ¼ cup of water

- 2 eggs

- 1 tbsp of oil (or maple syrup)

- 1 tsp of blue spirulina

- 1 tbsp of chia seeds

- Blueberries to taste

Instructions

1. Mix all ingredients in a blender

2. Add oil or butter to a pan

3. Pour desired amount of batter onto the pan

4. Add blueberries

5. Flip pancake

6. Cook until golden brown

7. Eat while it's hot!

Mushroom and kidney bean pattie

Prepartion time

35 minutes

INGREDIENTS

- 1 medium sweet potato

- 2 large Portobello/Field mushrooms

- Extra virgin olive oil

- 1 cup of cooked kidney beans

- 1 small carrot, roughly chopped

- 1/4 medium onion, roughly chopped

- 1 bunch fresh coriander, roughly chopped

- Breadcrumbs

- 1 teaspoon fresh chili (optional)

- 1 teaspoon ground cumin

- 1 egg

- Salad to serve (sliced tomato, lettuce leaves)

Instructions

1. Peel and cut the sweet potato into battens or chips – 2cm x 8cm.

2. Place on a baking tray with non-stick paper.

3. Remove mushroom stalks, place on the same baking tray and drizzle with extra virgin olive oil.

4. Roast in a 200ºC (392ºF) oven for 20 minutes, or until mushrooms and sweet potato are cooked.

5. In a food processor combine kidney beans, carrot, onion, coriander, breadcrumbs and spices.

6. Process to a rough paste.

7. Transfer to a bowl and mix through the egg.

8. Form into 2 patties.

9. Fry the patties in extra virgin olive oil until warmed through and browned on the outside.

10. To assemble, place the salad on the bottom of the plate, then the patty, your favourite sauce or chutney and top with the roasted mushroom.

11. Serve with the sweet potato chips on the side

Lentil and Vegetable Penne pasta

Preparation time

35 minutes

INGREDIENTS

- 2 tablespoons extra virgin olive oil

- 3 small carrots, peeled, finely chopped

- 3 celery sticks, finely chopped

- 2 garlic cloves, thinly chopped

- 1 large brown onion, coarsely chopped

- 1 small red capsicum, finely chopped

- 10-12 button mushrooms, thinly chopped

- 225 grams cooked brown lentils

- 150 grams Passata

- 500 grams No added sugar pasta sauce

- 500 grams High fibre pasta – Penne

Instructions

1. Heat the extra virgin olive oil in a large heavy-based saucepan over medium heat.

2. Add celery, carrot, onion, garlic and cook until just tender.

3. Add lentils, capsicum and mushrooms and cook, until just tender.

4. Add Passata and pasta sauce, bring to the boil.

5. Reduce heat to medium-low and simmer for 20 minutes.

6. Meanwhile, bring a large pot of water to the boil over high heat.

7. Add the penne pasta and cook, stirring often, for 10-12 mins or until tender. Drain.

8. Divide penne among serving bowls.

9. Spoon over the sauce. Serve.

Creamy Spinach Sweet Potato Noodles With Cashew Sauce

Prepartion time

2 hours 25 minutes

INGREDIENTS

- 1 cup cashews

- 3/4 cup water (more for soaking)

- 1/2 teaspoon salt

- 1 clove garlic

- 1 tablespoon oil

- 4 large sweet potatoes, spiralized

- 2 cups baby spinach

- a handful of fresh basil leaves, chives, or other herbs

- salt and pepper to taste

- olive oil for drizzling

INSTRUCTIONS

1. Cover the cashews with water in a bowl and soak for 2 hours or so.

2. Drain and rinse thoroughly.

3. Place in a food processor or blender (I got better texture with the blender) and add the 3/4 cup water, salt, and garlic.

4. Puree until very smooth.

5. Heat the oil in a large skillet over high heat.

6. Add the sweet potatoes; toss in the pan for 6-7 minutes with tongs until tender-crisp.

7. Remove from heat and toss in the spinach – it should wilt pretty quickly.

8. Add half of the herbs and half of the sauce to the pan and toss to combine.

9. Add water if the mixture is too sticky.

10. Season generously with salt and pepper, drizzle with olive oil, and top with the remaining fresh herbs.

Beetroot and cashew puree

Prepartion time

45 minutes

INGREDIENTS

- 250 grams fresh Beetroot

- 60 grams unsalted Cashews

- Extra virgin Olive Oil

- Salt

- Pepper

Instructions

1. Place whole beetroots into the bottom level of a bench top or cooktop steamer.

2. Place cashews in the steaming basket above and cook until beetroot is tender.

3. Remove beetroot skins and place into the stick blender chopper/food processor along with

the steamed cashews, salt and pepper & a drizzle of olive oil then blitz until smooth. Note– when blitzing, stop regularly to scrape down the sides of the processor or chopping attachment, drizzle more olive oil if mixture appears too dry.

4. Pass mixture through a sieve to ensure all hard, grainy particles are removed.

5. Using a touch of lemon infused olive oil works very well in this recipe if you have it available.

Chocolate avocado mousse

Preparation time

1 hour 5 minutes

INGREDIENTS

- 2 large avocados

- 3 tbsp honey

- 1 tsp vanilla bean extract

- 40 grams cocoa powder

Instructions

1. Place avocado flesh into a food processor with the honey, vanilla bean extract and cacao powder.

2. Blend/process until silky and smooth.

3. Transfer into chosen serving dish/es and refrigerate for at least 1 hour before serving.

Roast pumpkin puree

Prepartion time

15 minutes

INGREDIENTS

- 500 grams butternut pumpkin

- Extra virgin olive oil

- Salt

- Pepper

Instructions

1. Chop pumpkin, removing skin and seeds, and place in a baking dish.

2. Drizzle with extra virgin olive oil, sprinkle of salt and pepper and place into the oven.

3. Once tender remove from the oven and transfer into a jug/beaker.

4. Use stick blender to puree until smooth.

Carrot & Miso Soup with Silken Tofu

Prepartion time

40 minutes

INGREDIENTS

- 1 kg Carrots Peeled & Chopped

- 1 large Onion Diced

- 1.5 tsp Grated Fresh Ginger

- 3 cloves Garlic Crushed

- 1 litre Vegetable Stock

- 4 tbsp White Miso

- 200gm Silken Tofu

- 2 tbsp Sesame Oil

- Salt

- Pepper

- Coconut cream & additional sesame oil for garnishing (or extra virgin olive oil)

Instructions

1. Sauté onions, garlic, ginger and carrots in sesame oil until onions are translucent.

2. Add in vegetable stock, cover and simmer for 30 minutes stirring occasionally.

3. Add in white miso and silken tofu and blend using your modification tool of choice, adding more stock or water as needed (or alternatively coconut cream.)

4. Add salt and pepper to taste.

Note – if requiring thickened fluids add in medically prescribed thickening agent during step 2.

5. Ladle into serving bowls and serve with a drizzle of sesame or extra virgin olive oil and a touch of coconut cream.

Choc Smoothies

Prepartion time

10 minutes

INGREDIENTS

- 150 ml unsweetened almond milk

- ½ avocado

- 3 fresh strawberries

- 1 teaspoon raw cacao powder

- 1½ teaspoon natvia (natural sweetener)

- Ice to serve

Instructions

1. Combine almond milk, avocado flesh, strawberries, cacao and natvia in a blender.

2. Blend until smooth.

3. Serve in a glass with ice.

Apple Crumble Squares

Preparation time

1 hour 5 minutes

Ingredients:

- 1½ cups (375 mL) All-purpose flour

- 1 tsp (5 mL) Baking powder

- 1 tsp (5 mL) Cinnamon

- ½ tsp (2 mL) Salt

- ½ cup (125 mL) Sugar

- ½ cup (125 mL) Brown sugar, loosely packed

- 2 each Eggs

- ⅓ cup (75 mL) Vegetable oil

- 1 tsp (5 mL) Vanilla extract

- 4 cups (1 L) McIntosh apples, unpeeled, cored and ½ in. diced

Instructions

1. Preheat oven to 350°F (180°C). Line a 9 x 13 in. (3.5 L) pan with parchment paper and set aside.

2. Sift flour, baking powder, cinnamon, and salt together in a medium bowl and set aside.

3. In a large bowl, whisk together sugar, brown sugar, eggs, vegetable oil and vanilla extract until smooth.

4. Mix dry ingredients into wet ingredients until just incorporated.

5. Fold apples into the batter and spread evenly with spatula onto lined baking pan.

6. To prepare topping, place the ingredients in a medium bowl and gently rub together with fingertips until crumbly.

7. Top batter with crumb topping, and bake for 45-55 minutes.

8. Cake is ready when an inserted toothpick comes out clean.

Chocolate & Orange Date Cake

Preparation time

35 minutes

Ingredients:

- 1¾ cup (425 mL) Dried dates, pitted and chopped

- ⅓ cup (75 mL) Maple syrup

- 1 each Orange zest

- ¾ cup (175 mL) Water

- ½ cup (125 mL) Butter, room temperature

- ½ cup (125 mL) Sugar

- 1½ cup (375 mL) Tapioca flour

- ½ cup (125 mL) Cocoa powder

- ¼ tsp (1 mL) Baking soda

- Pinch Salt

- 3 tbsp (45 mL) Almond milk

Instructions

1. Preheat oven to 350°F (180°C).

2. Line 8 in. (2L) square pan with parchment paper and set aside.

3. In a sauce pan combine the dates, maple syrup, orange zest and water.

4. Simmer until mixture thickens to a jam consistency, approximately 15 minutes.

5. In a large mixing bowl, cream together butter and sugar and set aside.

6. In a separate bowl combine the tapioca flour, cocoa powder, baking soda and salt.

7. Stir to combine.

8. Mix dry ingredients into the butter and sugar. Stir in the thickened cooked dates and almond milk.

9. Spread mixture into lined pan and bake for 30 to 35 minutes. Let cool completely before slicing.

Pina Colada Cupcakes

Preparation time

25 minutes

Ingredients

Cupcakes:

- 1¼ cup (300 mL) All-purpose flour

- ¼ cup (60 mL) Dried shredded coconut, unsweetened

- ½ cup (125 mL) Sugar

- ½ tsp (2 mL) Baking powder

- ½ tsp (2 mL) Baking soda

- ¼ tsp (1 mL) Salt

- ½ cup (125 mL) Coconut milk

- ¾ cup (175 mL) Crushed pineapple, canned and well drained. Reserve juice.

- ½ cup (125 mL) Pineapple juice, from drained pineapple

- ¼ cup (60 mL) Vegetable oil

- ½ tsp (2 mL) Vanilla extract

Coconut Glaze:

- 1 cup (250 mL) Confectioner's sugar

- 1 tbsp (15 mL) Butter, softened

- 3 tbsp (45 mL) Coconut milk

- 1 tsp (5 mL) Vanilla extract

Instructions

Cupcakes:

1. Preheat oven to 350°F (180°C).

2. Line cupcake pan with liners and set aside.

3. In a large bowl, combine flour, shredded coconut, sugar, baking powder, baking soda and salt.

4. In a separate bowl, whisk together coconut milk, pineapple juice, vegetable oil and vanilla extract.

5. Add wet ingredients to dry ingredients and stir to combine.

6. Lastly, gently stir in crushed pineapple until just incorporated.

7. Using an ice cream scoop, divide batter into lined pan.

8. Bake for 25-30 minutes or until inserted toothpick comes out clean.

9. Allow to cool in pan for 5 minutes, and then transfer to a wire rack to cool completely.

Coconut Glaze:

1. Whisk confectioner's sugar, butter, coconut milk and vanilla extract together until combined.

2. About 30 seconds.

3. When cupcakes are completely cooled, frost with 2 tsp (10 mL) of icing each.

Fruit Bars

Prepartion time

20 minutes

Ingredients:

Base:

- ¾ cup (175 mL) Rolled oats, large flakes

- ½ cup (125 mL) All-purpose flour

- ½ cup (125 mL) Tapioca flour

- ½ cup (125 mL) Brown sugar, loosely packed

- ½ cup (125 mL) Dried shredded coconut, unsweetened

- ½ cup (125 mL) Dried apricots, finely chopped

- ½ cup (125 mL) Dried cranberries, roughly chopped

- ½ cup (125 mL) Raisins

- ½ cup (125 mL) Butter, softened

Topping:

- ½ cup (125 mL) Semi-sweet chocolate

Instructions

1. Preheat oven to 350°F (180°C). Line an 8 in. (2L) square pan with parchment paper and set aside.

2. In a medium bowl, blend all the dry ingredients together with fingers. Add mixture to softened butter and continue mixing with fingers until crumbly.

3. Spread into the lined baking pan and pat down firmly.

4. Bake for 15 to 20 minutes. You will know bars are ready when they are golden brown on the top.

5. Remove from oven and let cool to room temperature for 15 minutes. Refrigerate for 15 minutes until it is cold.

6. Melt chocolate in microwave and let cool to room temperature.

7. Spread onto cold fruit bars with a rubber spatula and return to refrigerator until chocolate is set. Cut into 24 bars.

Banana Berry Smoothie

Preparation time

5 minutes

Ingredients:

- 2 cups (500 mL) Orange juice

- 2 each Banana, cut in half

- 2 cups (500 mL) Blueberries, frozen

- 1 cup (250 mL) Strawberries, frozen

- 2 tbsp (30 mL) Honey

Instructions

1. In a blender, purée all ingredients until smooth.

2. Pour into an airtight container and keep refrigerated.

Strawberry Mango Smoothie

Prepartion time

5 minutes

Ingredients:

- 2 cups (500 mL) Almond milk

- 1 each Banana, cut in half

- 2 cups (500 mL) Mango, frozen

- 2 cups (500 mL) Strawberries, frozen

- 2 tbsp (30 mL) Honey

Instructions

1. In a blender, purée all ingredients until smooth.

2. Pour into an airtight container and keep refrigerated.

Blueberry Pancakes

Preparation time

25 minutes

Ingredients:

- 1 cup (250 mL) Gluten free all-purpose flour

- 2 tsp (10 mL) Baking powder

- 1 tsp (5 mL) Xanthan gum (if your gluten free flour already contains xanthan gum, omit from recipe)

- 2 tbsp (30 mL) Sugar

- 1 each Egg

- 1 cup (250 mL) Almond milk

- 2 tbsp (30 mL) Vegetable oil

- 1 tsp (5 mL) Vanilla extract

- 1 each Lemon, zest and juice

- 1 cup (250 mL) Blueberries, fresh

- 2 tbsp (30 mL) Butter, melted

Instructions

1. In a medium bowl, whisk together the flour, baking powder, xanthan gum and sugar.

2. In a small bowl, mix egg, almond milk, vegetable oil, vanilla, lemon zest and juice.

3. Add wet ingredients to dry ingredients all at once and whisk until combined.

4. Stir in fresh blueberries

5. Heat non-stick skillet on medium-high heat and brush pan with a little melted butter.

6. Pour ¼ cup (60 mL) of batter onto frying pan and cook until bottom is brown and bubbles appear on top.

7. Flip pancake and cook for another 1-2 minutes until cooked through.

Zucchini & Chocolate Cranberry Muffins

Prepartion time

45 minutes

Ingredients:

- 1 ½ cup (375 mL) Gluten free all-purpose flour

- 2 tsp (10 mL) Baking powder

- ½ tsp (2 mL) Baking soda

- ¾ tsp (4 mL) Xanthan gum (If your flour contains xanthan gum, omit this extra xanthan gum.)

- ¼ cup (60 mL) Brown sugar

- ¾ cup (175 mL) Almond milk

- 2 tbsp (30 mL) Honey

- 1 each Egg

- 1 tsp (5 mL) Vanilla extract

- 1 cup (250 mL) Zucchini, finely grated

- 1 cup (250 mL) Dried cranberries

- ½ cup (125 mL) Dark chocolate chips

Instructions

1. Preheat oven to 375°F (190°C). Line muffin tins with paper muffin cups and set aside.

2. Melt butter in microwave and set aside to cool.

3. In a large bowl, combine flour, baking powder, baking soda, xanthan gum and sugar mix thoroughly.

4. In a separate bowl, mix the almond milk, egg, cooled butter and vanilla extract.

5. Mix wet ingredients into the dry ingredients until smooth.

6. Gently mix in the grated zucchini, cranberry, dark chocolate chips until just incorporated. Batter should be lumpy.

7. Divide the batter evenly among the muffin cups.

8. Bake for 25-30 minutes, until a toothpick inserted into the centre comes out clean, and muffins are lightly browned.

Roasted Potatoes & Tomatoes

Prepartion time

45 minutes

Ingredients:

- 1 tbsp (15 mL) Baking soda/li>

- 3 each Russet potatoes, ½ in. diced

- 1 tbsp (15 mL) Paprika

- 1 tsp (5 mL) Salt

- 1 tbsp (15 mL) Olive oil

- 1 each Red pepper, thinly sliced

- 1 each Red onion, thinly sliced

- 1 pint Cherry tomatoes, cut in half

- 3 sprigs Basil leaves, chopped

- To taste Salt and pepper

Instructions

1. Preheat oven to 475°F (240°C).

2. Line a large baking tray with parchment paper and set aside.

3. Bring a large pot of water to boil. Add baking soda and potatoes to the boiling water.

4. Allow water to return to a boil and cook for 2 minutes.

5. Drain potatoes and transfer to a mixing bowl.

6. Add paprika, salt and 1 tbsp (15 mL) olive oil. Mix until potatoes are evenly coated.

7. Toss potatoes with peppers and onions and place onto the prepared baking tray.

8. Bake for 10 minutes, flip potatoes using a spatula and return to oven for another 15 minutes

9. You will know that they are finished when you can stick a knife into the potatoes very easily.

10. Season with salt and pepper.

11. Mix tomatoes and basil together with remaining olive oil.

12. Season with salt and pepper and serve with roasted potatoes.

Ginger & Veg Stir-Fry

Prepartion time

35 minutes

Ingredients:

- 125 g (⅓ pkg) Rice noodles, wide

- 1 tbsp (15 mL) Cornstarch

- ¼ cup (60 mL) Vegetable oil

- 2 cups (500 mL) Broccoli florets, bite-sized

- 1 each Carrot, thinly sliced half-moon shape

- 1 pkg (226 g) Mushrooms, quartered

- 1 each Red pepper, thinly sliced

- 1 each Yellow pepper, thinly sliced

- ½ cup (125 mL) Snow peas, stem removed

- 1 each Onion, sliced

- 1 clove Garlic, grated

- 2 tsp (10 mL) Ginger, grated

- 3 tbsp (45 mL) Soy sauce, light

- 3 tbsp (45 mL) Water

- ½ tsp (2 mL) Salt

Instructions

1. Bring a large pot of water to a boil and remove from heat.

2. Put rice noodles into pot and soak until they are al dente (approximately 20-25 minutes).

3. Check noodles periodically to make sure they do not become too soft.

4. When noodles are al dente, rinse with cold water and drain. Set aside.

5. In a large bowl, mix cornstarch and 2 tbsp (30 mL) of vegetable oil together until cornstarch is dissolved.

6. Toss broccoli, carrots, mushrooms, red pepper, yellow pepper and snow peas in cornstarch mixture to coat.

7. Heat the remaining oil, 2 tbsp (30 mL), in a large wok over medium high heat.

8. Sauté onions, garlic and ginger with oil.

9. Add vegetables and cook for 2 minutes, stirring constantly to prevent burning.

10. Mix soy sauce, water and salt together and add to the wok.

11. Add soaked rice noodles and gently stir fry until vegetables are cooked and tender.

12. Do not over mix.

Potato & Mushroom Pie

Prepartion time

1 hour 10 minutes

Ingredients:

- ½ each Potato, peeled and parboiled, ½ in. diced

- 2 tbsp (30 mL) Vegetable oil

- 1 each Onion, ½ in. diced

- 1 clove Garlic, minced

- ½ tsp (2 mL) Rosemary, dried

- 1 tsp (5 mL) Thyme, dried

- 1 cup (250 mL) Mushrooms, ½ in. diced

- ½ each Sweet potato, peeled and coarsely grated

- 1 tbsp (15 mL) Lemon juice

- To taste Salt and pepper

- 3 tbsp (45 mL) Butter

- 4 sheets Phyllo pastry

Instructions

1. Preheat oven to 375°F (190°C).

2. In a medium pot, bring 2 cups (500 mL) of water to a boil and add diced potatoes.

3. Return to a boil and cook for 2 minutes. Drain potatoes, run under cold water and set aside.

4. Heat oil in large skillet and add onions, garlic, rosemary and thyme.

5. Cook until onions become translucent and add potatoes.

6. When potatoes are golden, stir in the grated sweet potato, 1 tbsp (15 mL) of butter and mushrooms. Cook until mushrooms are tender and add lemon juice.

7. Season with salt and pepper and allow filling to cool.

8. Melt the remaining butter and set aside.

9. Lay 1 sheet of phyllo dough onto a clean cutting board and brush the entire surface with melted butter. Place another sheet of phyllo dough on top.

10. Cut into 6 equal pieces. Repeat this step with remaining 2 sheets of dough.

11. Line a standard size non-stick muffin tin with the phyllo squares allowing sides to hang over.

12. Place approximately ⅓ cup (75 mL) of filling into each muffin cup and fold hanging dough over to seal the pies.

13. Brush with remaining butter and bake for 15 minutes or until the pies are flaky and golden brown.

14. Gently remove from muffin tins and allow to cool on wire rack.

Veg Medley Stew

Preparation time

1 hour 5 minutes

Ingredients:

- ¼ cup (60 mL) Butter

- 1 each Onion, diced

- 3 each Garlic, minced

- 1 tsp (5 mL) Thyme, dried

- 1 tbsp (15 mL) Tomato paste

- ½ each Cauliflower, roughly chopped

- 3 cups (750 mL) Vegetable broth, low sodium

- 2 each Carrot, diced

- 1 each Red bell pepper, diced

- 2 each Zucchini, diced

- 1 can (796 mL) Diced canned tomatoes, with juices

- 1 tsp (5 mL) Salt

- ¼ tsp (1 mL) Black pepper

Instructions

1. In a large stockpot, heat 2 tbsp (30 mL) of butter.

2. Add onions, garlic, tomato paste and thyme.

3. Cook over a low heat, stirring occasionally, until onions are transparent.

4. Add in cauliflower and 2 cups (500 mL) of stock.

5. Bring to a boil and cook for approximately 5 minutes, until cauliflower is soft.

6. Purée with hand blender until smooth.

7. Heat remaining 2 tbsp (30 mL) of butter in a large sauté pan and add carrots.

8. Cook for 2 minutes and add red bell pepper.

9. Cook until carrots and peppers are caramelized.

10. Stir carrots and peppers into cauliflower purée along with zucchini and diced tomatoes. Bring to a boil.

11. Add remaining stock and salt and pepper.

12. Return to a boil and reduce to a simmer.

13. Cook for 20 minutes uncovered on a medium heat until stew has thickened. Season to taste.

Onion Gravy

Preparation time

35 minutes

Ingredients:

- 1 tbsp (15 mL) Butter

- 1 tbsp (15 mL) Vegetable oil

- 2 each Onions, finely chopped

- 1 tsp (5 mL) Sugar

- 1 tsp (5 mL) Red wine vinegar

- 2 cups (500 mL) Vegetable stock

- 1 tbsp (15 mL) Dijon mustard

- 1 pinch Black pepper

- To taste Salt

Instructions

1. In a small sauce pot on low heat, melt butter and add the vegetable oil.

2. Add onions and cook on low heat until they are browned and soft.

3. Approximately 20 minutes.

4. Add sugar and cook for 2 minutes.

5. Stir in vinegar and stock and cook for an additional 10 minutes or until gravy has reduced by half.

6. Stir in mustard and pepper.

7. Season to taste with salt.

8. Remove from heat and using a hand blender, blend until smooth.

Spicy Ketchup

Preparation time

35 minutes

Ingredients:

- 2 tbsp (30 mL) Vegetable oil

- 1 each Onion, diced

- 4 cloves Garlic, minced

- 1 each Red bell pepper, diced

- ½ cup (125 mL) Tomato paste

- 1 tsp (5 mL) Chili flakes, dried

- 2 tbsp (30 mL) Red wine vinegar

- ¼ cup (60 mL) Brown sugar, packed

- 2 tsp (10 mL) Salt

- 1 tsp (5 mL) Black pepper

Instructions

1. Heat oil in a small pot. Cook onions, garlic and red bell pepper until onions are caramelized on a

low heat for 10 minutes, stirring often to prevent burning.

2. Stir in tomato paste, chili flakes, vinegar and sugar.

3. Cook for an additional 10 minutes.

4. Remove pot from stove and purée using a hand blender.

5. Season with salt and pepper.

Tartar Sauce

Prepartion time

5 minutes

Ingredients:

- ¾ cup (175 mL) Mayonnaise

- ¼ cup (60 mL) Relish

- 1 tbsp (15 mL) Lemon juice

- 2 tbsp (30 mL) Green onion, chopped

- ¼ tsp (1 mL) Cayenne pepper (optional)

- 1 tsp (5 mL) Onion powder

- 1 each Lemon, zest and juice

- 1 each Egg

- 1 can (540 mL) Black beans, drained and rinsed

- 3 -213g cans Salmon, drained

- ½ cup (125 mL) All-purpose flour

- ¼ cup (60 mL) Vegetable oil

Instructions

1. Combine all ingredients and mix well.

2. Refrigerate in an airtight container until ready to serve.

Salmon Fish Cakes

Prepartion time

50 minutes

Ingredients:

- 4 each Green onion, chopped

- 1 tbsp (15 mL) Dried dill

- ¼ tsp (1 mL) Salt

- ¼ tsp (1 mL) Black pepper

- ½ tsp (2 mL) Cayenne pepper (optional)

- 1 tsp (5 mL) Onion powder

- 1 each Lemon, zest and juice

- 1 each Egg

- 1 can (540 mL) Black beans, drained and rinsed

- 3 -213g cans Salmon, drained

- ½ cup (125 mL) All-purpose flour

- ¼ cup (60 mL) Vegetable oil

Instructions

1. Combine green onion, dill, salt, black pepper, cayenne pepper, onion powder, lemon zest and juice, and egg in a medium bowl.

2. Mix until well combined.

3. Using a fork, slightly mash beans in a small bowl and add to egg mixture.

4. Flake salmon into large pieces with a fork. Incorporate into bean and egg mixture.

5. Add in ¼ cup (60 mL) flour and stir until combined.

6. Form into 8 cakes. Approximately ½ cup (125 mL) - ¾ cup (175 mL) of the mixture for each cake.

7. Gently press together to hold and dust cakes with remaining flour.

8. Heat half the vegetable oil, 2 tbsp (30 mL) in fry pan over medium heat.

9. Bake for 10 minutes, flip potatoes using a spatula and return to oven for another 15 minutes

10. Place fish cakes in heated pan and cook for 4 minutes.

11. Gently flip and cook for an additional 5 minutes or until the internal temperature reaches 160°F (71°C).

Southwestern-style Chicken & Quinoa

Prepartion time

1 hour

Ingredients:

- 4 each Chicken breasts, boneless and skinless

- ¾ tsp (4 mL) Salt

- ¼ tsp (1 mL) Black pepper

- Pinch Paprika

- 1 tbsp (15 mL) Garlic powder

- ⅓ cup (75 mL) Lime juice, reserve 2 tbsp (30mL) for dressing

- 2 tbsp (30 mL) Olive oil, reserve 1 tbsp (15 mL) for dressing

- 1 cup (250 mL) Quinoa

- ½ cup (125 mL) Monterey Jack cheese, grated

- 4 each Green onion, chopped

- ¾ cup (175 mL) Corn, canned and drained

- ¾ cup (175 mL) Black beans, canned and drained

- 2 each Plum tomatoes, seeded, ½ in. diced

Instructions

1. Preheat oven to 350°F (180°C).

2. Season chicken breast with salt, black pepper, paprika, garlic powder, 3 tbsp (45 mL) lime juice and 1 tbsp (15 mL) olive oil.

3. Transfer to baking dish and place in preheated oven. .

4. Rinse quinoa under running water for 3 minutes using a fine mesh sieve.

5. Cook quinoa according to package instructions.

6. Once quinoa is cooked let rest, uncovered.

7. After 15 minutes of cooking, turn over chicken and continue to cook for an additional 10 minutes.

8. After 10 minutes, sprinkle chicken breasts with grated cheese and return to oven for an additional 3 minutes, or until cheese is melted.

9. Remove from oven and cut into ½ in. slices.

10. Add ½ cup (125 mL) green onions, corn, black beans, and tomatoes to cooked quinoa.

11. Drizzle remaining 2 tbsp (30 mL) lime juice and 1 tbsp (15 mL) olive oil over quinoa. Season to taste with salt and toss to coat.

12. Use remaining green onions as a garnish.

Veg Chili

Prepartion time

40 minutes

Ingredients:

- 1 each Onion, chopped

- 4 cloves Garlic, minced

- 1 tbsp (15 mL) Vegetable oil

- 1 can (540 mL) Bean medley, canned, rinsed

- 1 can (796 mL) Diced canned tomatoes, with juices

- 1 cup (250 mL) Corn, frozen

- 1 each Lime, juiced

- 2 tbsp (30 mL) Chili powder

- 1 each Jalapeño pepper, seeded, diced (optional)

- 2 tsp (10 mL) Paprika powder

- 1 tsp (5 mL) Salt

- 2 cups (500 mL) Tomato juice

- 1 ½ cups (375 mL) Textured vegetable protein

- 4 pieces Green onion, chopped

Instructions

1. In a large pot, sauté the onions and garlic in vegetable oil until translucent.

2. Add beans, tomatoes, corn, lime juice, chili powder, jalapeño, paprika, salt and tomato juice. Mix thoroughly.

3. Cover pot and bring to a boil. Stir and reduce heat to a simmer.

4. Simmer while covered for about 20 minutes

5. Stir in textured vegetable protein and allow to cook for 3 – 5 more minutes.

6. Season to taste.

7. An additional ½ cup (125 mL) of water can be added if chili is too thick.

8. Stir in green onion. Season to taste.

MAPLE AND TAMARI GLAZED SALMON

Prepartion time

30 minutes

Ingredients

- Four 6-oz salmon fillets

- 1 tsp each salt and pepper

- 1 Tbsp olive oil

- 1/2 yellow onion cut into strips

- 1/4 cup pure maple syrup

- 2 Tbsp gluten-free tamari sauce

Instructions

1. Preheat the oven to 350 degrees.

2. Season salmon fillets on the top and sides with salt and pepper.

3. Heat olive oil in a large ovenproof skillet.

4. Add onion and sauté quickly over medium heat until it begins to darken and soften, approximately 4 minutes.

5. Push onion to one side and add salmon fillets, skin side up.

6. Sear 2 minutes undisturbed.

7. Turn fillets, drizzle with maple syrup and tamari, and finish in the oven until the internal temperature reaches 145 degrees, approximately 8 minutes.

8. Plate with onions and drizzle with pan sauce.

SUPERFOOD BUDDHA BOWL

Prepartion time

Ingredients For the turmeric quinoa:

- 1 cup quinoa

- 2 cups water

- 1 tsp dried turmeric

- 1 tsp curry powder

- 1/4 tsp salt

For the toasted chickpeas:

- 1 can of chickpeas, drained and rinsed

- 1 Tbsp olive oil

- 1 tsp cumin

- pinch cayenne, salt, and pepper

For the maple tahini sauce:

- 1/2 cup tahini

- 2 Tbsp maple syrup

- 2 Tbsp lemon juice

- 1/2 tsp cumin pinch cayenne

- 1/4 cup hot water (as needed to thin)

For the roasted vegetables:

- 1/2 lb broccoli florets

- 2 sweet potatoes, washed and chunked (bite-sized)

- 2 Tbsp olive oil

- pinch salt and pepper

Instructions

Make the turmeric tri-color quinoa:

1. Combine quinoa, water, turmeric, curry powder and salt and bring to a boil.

2. Cover and reduce heat to low.

3. Cook 15 min until liquid is absorbed.

4. Remove from heat and let rest 5 min before serving.

Make the maple tahini sauce:

1. Combine tahini, maple syrup, lemon juice, cumin and cayenne.

2. Add water a little at a time until a pourable consistency is reached.

3. Taste and adjust seasonings as desired.

Make the toasted chickpeas:

1. Combine chickpeas, olive oil, cumin, cayenne, salt and pepper

2. Spread on sheet pan and bake at 350 degrees for 10 min, toss and continue baking until crisp, approx. 5 min more.

3. Toss with a drizzle of olive oil and more salt/pepper/cayenne/cumin to reach desired taste.

Make the roasted vegetables:

1. Toss broccoli, sweet potatoes, olive oil, salt and pepper to combine.

2. Spread potatoes on parchment-lined sheet pan and roast at 350 degrees until softened, approx. 20 min.

3. Add broccoli and cook 8-10 min more.

4. Layer the quinoa, veggies, and chickpeas in bowl and drizzle with the maple tahini sauce.

Made in the USA
Las Vegas, NV
17 January 2022

41665327R00098